Run to You

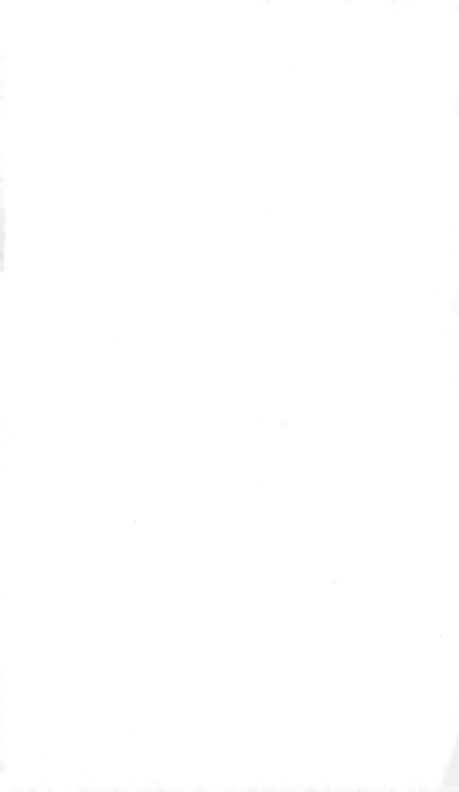

Run to You

a guide through
miscarriage

sarah siu

TATE PUBLISHING & Enterprises

Published by Tate Publishing & Enterprises, LLC
127 E. Trade Center Terrace | Mustang, Oklahoma 73064 USA

1.888.361.9473 | www.tatepublishing.com

Tate Publishing is committed to excellence in the publishing industry. The company reflects the philosophy established by the founders, based on Psalm 68:11,
"The Lord gave the word and great was the company of those who published it."

Book design copyright © 2007 by Tate Publishing, LLC. All rights reserved.
Cover design by Brandon Wood
Interior design by Kandi Evans

Published in the United States of America

ISBN: 978-1-60462-106-8

1. Christian Living, Practical Life   2. Miscarriage, Health, Women
07.09.13

Dedication

To April and Dr. John Brangenberg
who taught me the concept of running to God.

To Matthew and Anna
who brought me the opportunity
to run to Him in my
times of affliction.

Table of Contents

Foreword

Every major life crisis is a turning point, whether it is sickness, danger or loss from physical disasters, war, threats, physical attack, loss of job, home, or loved ones. We can either chose to run away from God in anger, disbelief, pain, shock, and blame, or run to God with all our anger, fear, hurt, frustration, burdens, pain, and blame, crying out for answers, help, and relief.

The first path only adds to the devastation of the crisis moment, because we have removed ourselves from our only hope, our only true source of relief and refuge. The second path ultimately leads to a deepening of our faith, hope, and trust in God, and becomes the foundation for rebuilding our broken lives.

At the beginning of the book of Job, Satan challenges God to test the quality of Job's commitment to God, asserting that anyone can be a loyal servant of God when life is all good. So God allows Satan to test Job. Job loses everything, his home, his flocks and herds, and all of his children. Then he is afflicted with painful boils from head to toe. If that is not bad enough, he has to endure the questioning and accusations of his three best friends who are trying to make sense of why this has happened to him, and try to defend himself against their indictments. He even has to endure the railings of a self-righteous young bystander who invents all sorts of evils that Job must have committed in order to incur the wrath of God with such magnitude. With nowhere else to turn, Job begins to lift up an outcry to God himself, confronting God with the injustice that he has suffered, challenging God to explain his actions toward Job. Suddenly God begins to speak to Job out of a whirlwind. He doesn't answer any of Job's questions or accusations. Rather He confronts Job with His presence. And healing and restoration begin.

Job has stumbled upon the only path that can lead to a healthy resolution to crisis. A path also taken by the authors of the over forty Psalms of Lament and the author(s) of the five laments in the book of Lamentations. He ran to God.

Choosing the path of running to God is not easy for us. It is so contrary to our innate instinct to cut and run. For many of us, we may first find ourselves naturally running away from God in those moments of crisis. But, if life is to go on with any sense of meaning and purpose or quality of life, we must come to a point of stopping in our tracks, turning around, and running back into the waiting arms of God.

In *Run to You,* the author, Sarah Siu, holds out her hand and offers to run with you as you run to God. You don't have to run this path alone. It is one that she has walked and run often. It is a path that is well worn in her heart and life. Sarah will help you to recognize the voice and the heart of God so that you, too, can turn and run to Him. Know, too, that even as you are running to God, He is running to you—and with you.

In the chapters that follow, Sarah lays out a path for running to God in one of the most difficult crises a couple can ever face, the loss of hope, dreams, and future that comes with the crushing experience of miscarriage. It is a path that my wife, April, and I walked through when we lost our first and only child to the devastating disappointment of miscarriage. It is a path that April and I walked together twice with Sarah and her husband, Koa, as they were eager newlywed students in my classes at Pacific Rim Bible College.

Sarah began writing this book immediately after she experienced her first miscarriage as a journal of her spiritual journey through this very difficult time in her life. It continued to grow as she retraced her steps after her second miscarriage. Sarah gave me a copy of her first draft back in 2002. Since then, Sarah has continued to reflect on what she experienced and learned as she and Koa sought refuge and comfort in the arms of God. Over those years, Sarah has grown and matured in wisdom and character into a wonderful minister, loving wife, caring mother, and radiant woman of God. And *Run to You* has grown to more than twice its original length as she has mined the riches of her journey with God into healing, courage, and restoration.

In this book, those who are struggling and suffering through the loss of miscarriage will find a gentle and wise guide through the process of rebuilding and renewing their lives together in the loving and comforting arms of God. The Father gently beckons, arms outstretched, waiting for you to make the choice that will change and renew your life, saying, "Run to me!"

"Cast your cares on the Lord and He will sustain you."
Psalm 55:22 NIV

Dr. John Brangenberg
Professor of Bible and Biblical Languages
Pacific Rim Bible College
Honolulu, Hawaii

Introduction

It was Christmas time and I was delighted to realize I was pregnant. *What a wonderful Christmas gift,* I thought. My husband and I were filled with joy. Bursting with excitement, we drove to my mother-in-law's house to share the news. She was thrilled. She couldn't wait to be a grandmother. Even before we were married, she would pick up things here and there for her future grandchildren. She started a whole collection of "baby treasures" in anticipation of us to have a baby. She was doubly thrilled that we told her we were pregnant on her birthday.

A new expectancy swept over me. I was going to be a mother. I was a mother. There was someone growing inside of me. I was in awe of this little miracle. I gathered books upon books about pregnancy, not to mention the books people gave me. I would look at pictures daily to see each stage of this little miracle.

"How big is he/she today? The spine is being formed as I speak." Thoughts of this nature ran through my mind almost all day. I was so happy to be pregnant. I was falling in love with the little one who was living and growing inside of me. *This is my baby,* I'd think.

Some weeks passed. I began to bleed. I clothed myself with prayer and invited people to pray over me. I went to the doctor. When it became a little more consistent, I decided to rest; and, as I did, I picked up a book called *How to Pray for Your Children.* I read about Hannah, a woman of God who pleaded for a child, and about how she dedicated her first child, the one she had fasted and prayed for, to the LORD. I thought, *I want that—I want all my children to be the Lord's.* I bowed my heart before the LORD and simply prayed that the child I carried would be His. I meant it with all my heart.

To my amazement, within the next twenty minutes I was rushed to the hospital's emergency room. Was He taking my baby now? I was scared to be there. All I could do was put my trust in the LORD. With tears in my eyes right there on the examination table, I began to sing, "Praise the name of Jesus, Praise the name of Jesus, You're my Rock, You're my Fortress, You're my Deliverer, In You will I trust."

I was shocked. I didn't believe what the doctor said. I had lost my baby. In one day, I went from mother to mourner. I had been hopeful. I had been trusting. Now I was broken.

My husband, Koa, and I thought that the baby we lost was a boy, so we named him Matthew.

Time went by. I got back into the routine of my life. Then, in October 2001 (shortly after the September 11th attack on the World Trade Center) I found myself pregnant again! I was overjoyed. Yet, in the depths of my heart, I was actually petrified as I pondered where this might lead. I did not want to get my hopes up. I took special care of myself and enjoyed every minute of my pregnancy. At first, we were reluctant to share our good news with others, but we did anyway, in hopes of receiving their prayers and support. Then it came so fast and sudden. The bleeding started again. It had only been a couple of weeks. I wept and wept. We decided to see the doctor and headed for the emergency room. I couldn't believe it was happening all over again.

The month that followed was long and hard. I found myself at the doctor's office frequently for blood tests, ultrasounds, and other tests. The doctors were concerned because my pregnancy hormone level did not drop fast enough, and this catapulted me on to an emotional roller-coaster ride, punctuated with invasive examinations.

Finally, all that I had written about the first miscarriage flooded across my emotions and into my mind. I had written about running to God. I remembered how He helped me through my previous loss and how He had comforted my aching heart. I had found peace and assurance in Him.

The morning after my first miscarriage, I knew that I stood at a crossroads. I found myself there again. It was a fork in the road of life. This was a place where I had to decide whether I was going to let this drive me away from God or push me closer to Him. Was I going to run to Him or away? This question was *the magnified question* in my mind and heart.

Was it going to happen again? I didn't want to think about it, but I couldn't escape the nagging fear. I did not want to be in this situation again, but I was. Denial wasn't going to change things. The baby was gone. I was left only with tears, grief, disappointment, and even anger.

Prior to this miscarriage, I thought this little miracle of life was a girl, so we named her Anna—a name that is dear to my heart. In my mind, my beautiful daughter has big eyes and brown hair. In reality, I have never seen her. But in her very unique DNA blueprint is the special person God created her to be. I venture to wonder what that blueprint contained. Did she have her father's eyes and my nose? God knows. He knit her together.

Time passed painfully. Deep down in my spirit I

knew that the only way to get through all of this was to run to Him—the only One who could heal me. No one else could satisfy or take away my pain. He alone could give me hope. I agonized over my decision. Who could I trust with my deepest disappointment? Finally, I made a conscious choice to run to Him no matter what. I would have to take Him at His word. This choice started me on the journey and ongoing action of running to Him.

I have found the words in this book to be helpful and comforting, and I hope they will be for you too. This book is dedicated to our son, Matthew, and daughter, Anna, who are now at home with their Father in heaven. By God's grace, they taught me what it means to run to the LORD.

Run to You

By Koa Siu

What can I say as the tears run down her face?

I've never been here before
Pieces of her heart lying broken on the floor
I've never been here before

I see her crying, lost in the feeling
And it's true, grief is rarely shared
Inside she's dying, and the pain she's feeling
Is more than I can know, and more than she can bear

She doesn't know what to do so she runs to You
(Jesus) You've been here before
Though her heart is lonely, it finds a friend in You
No matter what she's suffered, You've suffered more
You understand, so she opens up the door

What can I say, as the tears roll down my face
I've never been here before
Pieces of my heart, crushed and broken on the floor
I've never been here before

I sit here crying, lost in the feeling
Not ready yet for comfort but thankful that You care
Inside I'm dying, and the pain I'm feeling
Is deeper than I've ever known, and more than I can
bear

I don't know what to do so I run to You
(Jesus) You've been here before
Though my heart is lonely, it finds a friend in You
No matter what I've suffered, You've suffered more
You understand, so I open up the door

Download this song free of charge at
www.runtoyou.org.

Run To Him

While I was visiting my mother one Saturday morning, I saw a little girl wandering around. She was about three years old and was barefoot on the wet grass. She threw her hands up in the air and then she placed them restlessly between her curly locks. "Daddy...Daddy? Where are you?" she repeated.

I said to her, "Are you lost?"

She said, "No, I'm looking for my daddy!"

I said to myself, *That's me.* I just wanted my daddy. I needed my daddy.

I watched her carry on until finally she saw her father. She ran over to him. She didn't hesitate. She held nothing back. He greeted her with love and swept her off the ground. I watched him hold her in his arms as he strolled along. Later he set her feet on the ground and took her by the hand, and he did not let go. Running to the LORD is no different.

What Does it Mean to Run to Him?

Running to Him means not hesitating to open your heart to God. It means coming before Him in prayer—sometimes on your knees, sometimes shouting. It means being honest with Him to His face. It means persevering. It means not giving up on your faith in Him. It means drawing near to Him by being still in His presence. You can simply run to Him, by humbly kneeling and acknowledging He is real.

Running to Him means not seeking other things to fill our needs.

The little girl could have chosen instead to give up looking for her father. What if she went back to her house, locked her door, and curled up in a ball on her bed? What if instead of trying to find him, she ran the other way and shut herself off from him all together? She is a child. She has faith like a child! In the Gospel of (Luke 18:17), Jesus says, "Truly I say to you, whoever does not receive the Kingdom of God like a child will not enter at all." This saying is repeated in all the Synoptic Gospels. Jesus is making a point to his disciples: He's talking about simple faith. Running to Him—receiving the Kingdom—means we humble ourselves to think of him like a child thinks of her loving father. When a child gets hurt, she runs to her mommy or daddy. She does cry and is hurt, but something in her knows that her parent can change everything and make her better. Somewhere in the midst of becoming an "adult," we lose sight of this. We don't need to run to the LORD when we're hurt. "I'm an adult," we say. "I don't need God." But inside, when we come to the crossroads, we know we do.

Running Away

Once, a few years ago, I had a vision in which I saw myself looking and searching for something. I was going to the left and to the right wandering aimlessly. I had my hands out ready to grab whatever came around. All the while Jesus was walking behind me with His arms open waiting to embrace me. He was just waiting for me to turn. How could I deny myself the very thing I needed—Him! In scripture, I see that this happens over and over again.

In Luke 22, we see two key examples of people turning away from Jesus. Judas turned away from Jesus in Luke 22:4, "He went away and discussed with the chief priests and officers how he might betray Him to them." Judas went away. He left and turned from the very thing that he needed—Jesus. Again in Luke 22:55–62, Peter denies Jesus...not just once, but three times. He too had turned away from Jesus in His heart. He denied himself the very thing He needed—his relationship with Jesus. In vs. 62, Jesus looked at Peter and he wept bitterly. Jesus knew that Peter would deny Him. He even told Peter earlier that he would (vs. 34). Here we see Jesus knowing that these would turn away and yet He dines with them and invites them to remember Him. He does not force us to stay and love Him, but He waits for us to love Him. Jesus humbly allows us to make these choices.

This shows me that when I deny Him, I deny Him coming close to me. When I walk through life just like the vision described above, I need to turn around to the embracing arms of Jesus. He has known my turning and has still remained faithful. He is always there to run to. In my time of need instead of running *away* I desire to run *towards*. This isn't easy. We feel afraid that if we turn and embrace Him maybe he won't do the same. We think, *Will He leave? Will He deny me? Will He ever forgive me?* At these times we can hold on to His promise, "I will never desert you, nor will I ever forsake you" (Hebrews 13:5).

Draw Near

When we run to Him we are deciding to draw near to Him. Many times my husband wants to "connect" with me. When I'm having a bad day I honestly want to close myself off from him and everyone else. He desires intimacy, and I desire to run away! Drawing near is like letting down your guard and choosing to get closer. I need to choose to draw near as well as express it outwardly. If I just look at my husband and tell him, "I would like to draw near to you," but choose to stay in a different room for the rest of the night—I am not drawing near. Even though I might say it aloud my intentions and my actions need to line up with my decision to draw near.

Drawing near to God is like a deer that draws near to water. The deer in the forest longs for water and seeks out a stream. Once in view, the deer is drawn to it. The deer is compelled to drink knowing that the source is available now. Sometimes the deer needs to find a safe place to drink. There are rocks, waterfalls, other animals, and bushes with thorns. Most of all the deer doesn't want to be seen in broad daylight—afraid of man and afraid of so much. She chooses to go to the stream. She is defenseless and vulnerable. Yet she goes. And she drinks. She remains there until she is full.

The desire of our hearts determines whether or not we will choose to draw near. If we are willing and trusting, we can take the first steps. James writes, "Draw near to God and He will draw near to you" (James 4:8). God is right here waiting and longing to bring us near—if we are willing to come.

What does this look like practically?

The practical application of running to Him takes on many different forms for many different people. Finding what works the best for you (that doesn't include running away) is important.

1. *Find a place where you feel safe expressing yourself to God and run there! Find a place where you can be alone with Him and where you feel free to cry and simply "be." Some helpful places are: your bathroom, bedroom, a closet or spare room, and even an empty living room. The place may change, but it's important to find a place where you're not distracted and you're able to draw near to God. When you do, He will already be drawing near to you.*

2. *Kneel or fall on your face. I know many people say, "I've got knee problems" and so on. Just find a way to humble yourself and really connect. I find that getting on the floor sometimes is just the thing my spirit needs as an action of running to Him and expressing my need.*

3. *Pour out your heart. Say what's on your heart and mind. If you're mad, upset, or disappointed, tell Him.*

Let Him know how you feel. Let it out. This is a continuous process and journey of running to Him.

"Arise, cry aloud in the night at the beginning of the night watches; pour out your heart like water before the presence of the LORD; Lift up your hands to Him for the life of your little one." (Lamentations 2:19)

Grieve with Him

"Be gracious to me, O Lord, for I am in distress; my eye is wasted away from grief, my soul and my body also."
Psalm 31:9

When hit with loss, the massive amount of grief that comes can feel like a ton of bricks or a tsunami wave. Grief invites its friends—Distress, Sorrow, and Heartache—to move in and invade your entire mind, body, and soul.

To me, these were unwelcome guests. I wasn't a stranger to suffering. But loss was an intruder that barged in and turned everything upside down, leaving me sitting in an insurmountable pile of emotions. It was imperative that I process these emotions in God's presence. Learning to run to Him in the pain of grief and allowing Him to be with me through it was not easy. I didn't want to sit in grief. But it was brought to me. Grief's initial effect in my life was weeping.

Weep

"My soul weeps because of grief; strengthen me according to Your word."

Ps. 119:28

Thus says the LORD, "A voice is heard in Ramah, Lamentation and bitter weeping. Rachel is weeping for her children; She refuses to be comforted for her children, because they are no more." Thus says the LORD, "Restrain your voice from weeping and your eyes from tears;...there is hope for your future."

Jeremiah 31:15–17

Grief can cause weeping that is unexplainable. Throughout history people have wept over wars, loss of loved ones, endless years of oppression, injustice, and ill treatment. In the verses above God recognizes the loss that Israel is experiencing during the exile. This verse is also mentioned in the gospel of Matthew to depict the grief mothers felt when Herod slew all the male babies in Bethlehem.

I can't imagine what it was like for so many mothers to lose their sons. Was the weeping so loud it rang in the ears of the guards? Did it echo in the streets? Their loss seemed so great.

My loss seemed so small. Yet, especially when we experienced the first miscarriage, I needed time to weep. I remember my husband holding me as I wept. It was so hard to understand how I could have so much emotion over the loss of someone I'd never known. Yet I wept.

To make sense of the weeping I turned to God's Word. Scripture shares with us a vast amount of insight into what it means to weep. There is a time to weep (Ecc. 3:4). There are places to weep (Gen. 43:30). There are people to weep with (Rom. 12:15). Jesus Himself wept (John 11:35). It seems to be a natural response to grief and loss.

I used to joke with God about the promise, "You have taken account of my wanderings; *Put my tears in Your bottle.*" I'd tell Him, "You must have buckets up there for me…perhaps a swimming pool." This thought got me through moments where the tears just kept coming.

You may find your initial response to grief is to weep. Some may experience shock first. Whatever your response to grief, it will impact you mentally, spiritually, and physically. The good news is that you don't have to go through it alone.

Jesus

The example of suffering and running to the Father

"And He went a little beyond them and fell on His face
and prayed, saying, "My Father, if it is possible, let this
cup pass from Me; yet not as I will, but as You will."
Matthew 26:39

In the Garden of Gethsemane, Jesus came to the
Father. He fell on His face knowing the suffering He
would soon endure. His ultimate heartache would be
to be separated from the Father. He says, "My soul is
deeply grieved, to the point of death." He wasn't in
physical pain yet. He had pain in His heart and spirit
that He couldn't express in words. His expression took
the form of sweat like drops of blood. He came, He
knelt, and He fell on His face before His Abba. This
is the only place He could go, and He desired to go
there. This emotion could not be held in. This grief
was real. He truly knew sorrow and grief. Three times
He came to pray. I can imagine Him crying out.

In the pericope of the Garden of Gethsemane we see
Jesus as the obedient and sacrificial Savior. Jesus enters
Gethsemane. This is a familiar place to Him and His
disciples. They had often traveled there because it was
between two of Jesus' favorite places, a Sabbath day's

walk to Jerusalem and to Bethany. Also, it was a place of rest and prayer. He probably prayed there many times, but this time it was with so much more emotion.

Jesus is grieved to the point of death. He came falling on His face. Jesus didn't shy away from the Father. He didn't ignore His suffering. He didn't blame His Father. He came to Him intimately in prayer. Jesus was faced with a crisis and decided, "I am running to the Father."

Jesus is our example of running to the Father despite our grief. He knew who to cling to. He knew the only way to deal with such grief was by being on His face and pouring out His heart to the One who loves Him. It was not by suppressing the anguish and becoming bitter. It was not by getting angry with the Father. The way to deal with the grief was running to Him, to the only one who can truly strengthen, to Him who has restoration and healing for all.

We need to follow His example when we are crushed. By doing so we will find what we really need—and that's *Him*. Psalm 34:18 says, *"The Lord is near to the broken hearted, and saves those who are crushed in spirit."*

Lord, You are near to me when I cry about my loss. I grieve and mourn before you. I am hurt and broken. I need You and I need to come to You. Heal me, O Lord. Your Word says You are near to those who are brokenhearted. Please draw near to me. You are my answer, You are my hope, You are my life. I run to You, my Father.

Surrender

I once watched an Oprah show where two families were caught up in an adoption scandal. Both families claim to have adopted twin baby girls. The first family gave money to have the babies, and the birth mother was going to place them in their custody. But then she changed her mind. Her facilitator took the opportunity to gain money from another family. Both families paid and spent time doing the paper work. The whole situation spiraled into a big mess. Eventually, all the parties ended up in court. You can imagine the conflicting stories that were told. On top of it all, the birth mother was now pleading for her children back. The question arose, "Who do these babies really belong to?"

I asked myself this same question when I experienced my first miscarriage. God was calling me to let go of Matthew and entrust my son to Him. *But, isn't this* my *baby?* I'd think. *How can I let him go?* Even though Matthew was not here with me anymore, it was very hard to let go. The memories, the hopes, the dreams, the anticipation, all this needed to be surrendered. My right to be a mother needed to be surrendered. My baby's short life and little spirit needed to be surrendered.

In the presence of God's safe arms, I began to let go. It wasn't easy, but as I poured out my heart in trust to Him surrender seemed to follow. Surrender comes out of an open heart that is willing to trust. "Trust in him at all times, O people; pour out your hearts to him, for God is our refuge" (Psalm 62:8). The act of running to the LORD depends upon surrender. To get to a place of being on your knees, you must release your expectations and be willing to relinquish whatever may hold you back.

It's like a tree. The autumn trees display their leaves of so many beautiful colors. This breathtaking season is known for the leaves changing colors and falling to the ground—one leaf at a time. The branch knows it needs to let go of that little leaf, and it happens so graciously. The branch will soon be bare and empty, but it lets go anyway. The next season is right around the corner, but sometimes it's nearly impossible to see. Nevertheless, the branches let the leaves go.

Sometimes we need to learn how to be like a tree with branches that let its leaves go. We need to trust that our Creator will bring us into springtime after the harsh winter.

Tested to Surrender

Does God really want to test us by asking us to surrender? I think so. Does He really test us to surrender our children? I think so. There are many "tests" that characters in the Bible faced. The Israelites were tested in the wilderness, "You shall remember all the way which the LORD your God has led you in the wilderness these forty years, that He might humble you, *testing you,* to know what was in your heart, whether you would keep His commandments or not" (Deuteronomy 8:2, *emphasis mine*).

In Exodus 20:20, Moses encourages the people, "Do not be afraid; for God has come in order to test you, and in order that the fear of Him may remain with you, so that you may not sin." Israel was tested to see what was really in their hearts. The act of being tested is like shining a flashlight in the darkness of our hearts. The light is shed on whom and what we are really living for.

Abraham and Isaac

In the Old Testament (Genesis 22), Abraham was tested to see if he loved the LORD more than his own son. I know this sounds crazy, but Abraham actually almost killed his own son in obedience to God, and in so doing proved that he loved God more than anyone or anything. He literally was willing to let go of his son—his only true son. This was his heir. The one God promised to him. Through this son "all the nations of the earth shall be blessed" (Genesis 22:18). Abraham was tested, and he passed.

Abraham's story of sacrifice foreshadows God the Father giving His only begotten Son for us. In John 3:16 Jesus says, "For God so loved the world that He gave His only begotten Son, that whosoever believes in Him shall not perish but have eternal life." This verse gives me comfort because in it I realize that *God must know how I felt when I lost my son.* It also shows me that He loved me and gave His Son for me. After losing my own son, I can better identify with God the Father in His time of seeing Jesus die on the cross.

Jesus' life was surrendered in love for us. In the same way, we can trust him and emotionally let go of our loss.

When we are tested to surrender, we are tested to see "where our treasure is." "For where your treasure is there you heart will be also" (Matt. 6:21). What and whom do you love? What is your treasure? For me, it was my baby. I was tested to surrender and love the LORD above my son and daughter.

If we love others more than Jesus, we are not worthy of Jesus! This is what Jesus says in Matthew 10:37, "He who loves father or mother more than Me is not worthy of Me; and he who loves son or daughter more than Me is not worthy of Me." These certainly are intense words to receive.

When we are asked to surrender our loved ones, we are being asked, "Whom do we really love?" If we find that we can't love Jesus more than our relationships, we may have set those people as the treasure of our heart. This can easily become an idol or stronghold. An idol is anything we serve, worship, love, or live for more than and besides God. The greatest commandment is "You shall love the LORD your God with all your heart, with all your soul, and with all your strength, and with all your mind; and your neighbor as yourself."

As followers of Christ, we are called to live a radical life where Jesus is LORD over every aspect of our being forever! Jesus is worth more than life. Jesus is worth all of our love and adoration, more than any relationship here on earth. What would you surrender to love Him who is most worthy?

Surrender Out of Love and Trust in the Lord

Surrender comes out of love and trust. If you truly love God, there is nothing you would withhold from Him and no one you would love more. He is the costly pearl that a merchant would sell everything and give all that he had to obtain.

The woman in Luke 7:36 came to Jesus and poured out upon His precious feet all that she had. She held in her hand and alabaster flask filled with expensive perfume oil. It was so valuable people didn't understand why she would extravagantly pour it out on His feet. *If she wanted to give it to the cause,* they thought, *she should have kept the perfume in the bottle. We could have sold it and fed the poor. What a waste!*

But she wasn't giving it to the "cause," she was simply loving her Lord—she was surrendering her life. Out of sheer love for Jesus, she surrendered all she had. She broke her alabaster flask and poured it out before Him. She did it while kissing and weeping at His feet. She found someone worth more than that priceless alabaster flask. Her love was displayed in her willingness to surrender it all and pour it out unto Jesus.

The Example of Hannah

Now there was a certain man...his name was...Elkanah...He had two wives: The name of one was Hannah and the name of the other Peninnah; and Peninnah had children, but Hannah had no children. Now this man would go up from his city yearly to worship and to sacrifice to the LORD of hosts in Shiloh...When the day came that Elkanah sacrificed, he would give portions to Peninnah and his wife and to all her sons and her daughters; but to Hannah he would give a double portion, for he loved Hannah, but the LORD had closed her womb. Her rival would provoke her bitterly to irritate her, because the LORD has closed her womb. It happened that year after year, as often as she went up to the LORD she would provoke her; so she wept and would not eat. Then Elkanah her husband said to her, "Hannah, why do you weep and why do you not eat and why is your heart sad? Am I not better to you than ten sons?" Then Hannah rose after eating and drinking in Shiloh. Now Eli the priest was sitting on the seat by the doorposts of the temple of the LORD. *She, greatly distressed, prayed to the Lord and wept bitterly.* She made a vow and said, "O Lᴏʀᴅ of hosts, if You will indeed look on the affliction of Your maidservant and remember me, and not forget Your maidservant, but will give Your maidservant a son, then I will give him to the Lᴏʀᴅ all the days of his life, and a razor shall not come on his head." Now it came about, as she continued praying before the Lᴏʀᴅ, that Eli was watching her mouth. As for Hannah, she was speaking in her heart, only her lips were moving, but her voice was not heard. So Eli thought she was drunk. Then Eli said to her, "How long will you make yourself drunk? Put away your wine from you." Hannah replied, "No, my Lᴏʀᴅ, *I am a woman oppressed in spirit;* I have drunk neither wine nor strong drink, *but I have poured out my heart before the Lord.* Do not consider your maidservant as a worthless woman, for I have spoken until now out of my great concern and provocation." Then Eli answered and said, "Go in peace; and may the God of Israel grant your petition that you have asked of Him." She said, "Let your maidservant find favor in your sight." So the woman went her way and ate, and *her face was no longer sad.*

1 Sam. 1:1–18

Can You Relate?

When I read about Hannah, I relate with her sufferings. I also learn a lot from her example of pouring out her heart to God. She could easily have never prayed again. She could have cursed God and disregarded Him completely. Instead, she opens up to Him. I hope that you can relate to Hannah.

Hannah and the Hard Reality

Hannah was faced with the hard reality that her womb was closed; she was barren. Wherever she went her rival would remind her. She couldn't run away from this issue that troubled her heart. She was provoked constantly. This is like being in immeasurable debt and receiving a bill everyday. You are constantly reminded of what you don't have. She was reminded of her emptiness probably everyday. Hannah was pushed and irritated.

When you first hear this or read this it seems awful. But, there is a blessing to be found. She was pushed to deal with her feelings instead of deny them. Because the issue of her barrenness was raised often, she had to wrestle with her heart. God sometimes brings these things up so that He can begin His good work in us. If she simply denied her feelings, she would have remained a bitter woman. She would not have ever asked for a child; she would have kept this all in her heart. Sometimes these painful reminders help us run to the LORD. These "bills" make us go to the bank. They're not always fun and "happy," but they bring us to deal with the hard reality and its emotional effect on our hearts.

Once your eyes are open to the reality and your spirit can agree that this is your situation, then you can bring it to the LORD for help.

When a child gets hurt, one of the first things she does is run to her parents. But do you remember that often when you get hurt as a child you don't realize it until you see the wound bleeding? Once you see it, indescribable pain comes upon you! The same thing applies to spiritual wounds: you have to see it first, feel its pain, and then that pain drives you all the more to find refuge in the Father.

She was Loved and Nurtured

Often, when we read about Hannah we focus on what she didn't have—a baby. But, if you look closer, you can find that God provided for her and blessed her despite her closed womb. She had a loving husband. God chose to love Hannah through her husband. He would give her a double portion. Her husband loved her enough to notice all that she was going through. He said to her, "Hannah, why do you weep and why do you not eat and why is your heart sad? Am I not better to you than ten sons?" (1 Sam. 1:8). He tried to comfort her and encourage her. It is easy to overlook those who are dearest to you when loss comes. Sadly, God chooses to love us through people that we unknowingly disregard. God sent love and encouragement through Hannah's husband and also through the priest, Eli. Eli sat and watched her at the temple. God placed him there to see Hannah and look upon all that she was going through. Often God sends us encouragement from friends at church that we will miss if we are not open to it.

Hannah was loved and tested to see what she really wanted. Would having children make her happy? Or would she be content with the love of just her husband? She chose a third option. She chose someone whom she could confide all things too.

She Poured Out Her Heart and Soul

Hannah openly and honestly prayed to the LORD. She didn't just cry a few drops. She wept. She wept so hard that she couldn't make sense. She wept so hard that no sound could come out of her mouth with the words. She spoke all that was bottled up from the many painful reminders. She brought her oppressed spirit before her LORD. She didn't keep pretending everything was all right. She cried out to God. She asked Him to look upon her affliction. Out of all of this, she was able to surrender to the LORD and ask for a son.

She Surrendered

Hannah surrendered by allowing the fate of having children to be in His hands. She came to a point when she said, "It's all up to You, LORD." She also went beyond that to surrender the very thing she was asking for. She would dedicate this son to the LORD forever. She did this spiritually, emotionally, and eventually physically. She gave Him the choice. She let God be God. She gave in to the reality and released the tension of her heart.

After she did this, the text says, "her face was no longer sad." God did something in her time of vulnerability. He changed her heart. He gave her contentment. She gave Him control, and He gave her peace.

Hope and trust came. Her longing was left in the arms of the Father, and in His due time—if it be His will—she would conceive.

Surrender is so hard to do because it feels like we're losing something so worthwhile and precious, and often, we are.

For me, surrendering Matthew and Anna didn't happen just once. I lost them. I surrendered them. Then a few days later, I'm walking through a mall and passing the baby store—and I have to lose them all over again. Day after day, I still need to entrust them to the LORD.

Lord, I want to pour out my heart to You.
I want to be free to weep in front of You.
Help me, Lord.
Help me surrender control to You.
It's hard to let my baby go.
It was hard then and it's hard now, in Your presence.
I entrust my baby to You.
Keep this child.
Help me to trust You.

Healing and Restoration

Healing and restoration occur in the presence of God. Simply by encountering His Spirit, we are touched in the core of our being. His Spirit brings comfort that was not there before. In His comfort, we are free to cry and safe to be vulnerable. It is when we run to Him that we find the healing that we need and that He longs to give. "Therefore the LORD longs to be gracious to you, and therefore He waits on high to have compassion on you" (Isaiah 30:18).

The first step to finding His healing and His presence is to ask for it. In the Old Testament, Jeremiah, a prophet surrounded by hardships and personal trials, cried out to LORD, "Heal me, O LORD, and I will be healed; save me and I will be saved, for You are my praise" (Jeremiah 17:14). If we do not ask for His healing, we may never experience it.

Jesus encouraged us to ask, "Until now you have asked for nothing in My name; ask and you will receive, so that your joy may be made full" (John 16:24). He is aware of our hurts and our emptiness. In this passage, He is encouraging His disciples that though they will be experiencing deep sorrow over His death, it will be turned to joy. Somehow, by seeking Him and asking Him, they would find joy.

Once we ask for healing, we need to receive it and allow Him to continue this work in us. Jesus came to bind up the brokenhearted (Isaiah 61), and He is still about this business today in our lives. "For I will restore you to health and I will heal you of your wounds,' declares the LORD" (Jeremiah 30:17). We have the choice to receive this healing and comfort or refuse it (Jeremiah 31:15). One outcome of refusing His comfort and grace is bitterness.

Bitterness

Bitterness is perhaps the biggest hindrance to healing and restoration. I find that bitterness is a direct result of unresolved pain. It is important to be honest before the LORD and weep before Him and confess when we are bitter. "See to it that no one comes short of the grace of God; that no root of bitterness springing up causes trouble and by it many be defiled" (Hebrews 12:15). This is not easy. The author of Hebrews describes bitterness like a root. Roots can extend quite a ways. They can go deep and in many directions. Uprooting them can be an endless headache. There is a possibility that the roots can grow back and create the same mess all over again. On our own, it is impossible to simply "not be bitter." You can't simply "ignore" roots. But in this passage it is His grace that uproots the tangled mess. His grace is like a healing salve that allows deep roots to slide out. Jesus describes Himself as a Physician, (Matthew 9:12, Luke 4:23). He is able, like a good surgeon, to remove a stubborn "shard of glass" or "deep root." But it takes coming to Him and allowing Him to operate.

Sometimes it can be hard to pin point, "Who or what am I really bitter at?" We can be bitter at loved ones, strangers, God, ourselves, and even our circumstances. But you can rest assure; the heart does know its own bitterness (Proverbs 14:10). Here is a simple prayer you can pray from the Psalms, "*Search me, O God, and know my heart; Try me and know my anxious thoughts; and see if there be any hurtful way in me, and lead me in the everlasting way*" (Psalm 139:23–24). In this passage, the psalmist David is asking God to reveal any hurtful ways in him. I find this prayer very effective in my life. God can reveal where the unresolved pain is coming from. It takes me a little while to break through my own denial to believe what He is really revealing. But like a good physician, I can trust He will find that spot and test it—revealing my weakness.

After I experienced my second miscarriage, I was pondering what hurt me most about my first miscarriage, and I think it was the hurt of an unmet expectation. One day I was a mother and the next I was not. My first miscarriage left me bitter at God. My second miscarriage left me bitter at the doctors and the endless testing. I was hurt that I could not escape the physical pain.

My pastor describes being bitter as drinking a vile of poison and waiting for the other person to die. In many cases, the other person is not going to be affected by *your* bitterness, but it will eat you up inside. Being bitter at God was not helping me in any way. In fact, it made things worse because He was the only one who could help me.

Though physically I was hurting, spiritually I had to learn to run to Him. Through His grace, I chose to draw close to him in the pain and bitterness. Through times of worship, soaking in the scriptures, and the healing power of God I began to heal. It helped to read about other Biblical characters that struggled with bitterness—Job, Isaiah, and Peter. It takes time to work through the bitterness and sort through the roots with God. But it is a process with a promise. *"He heals the brokenhearted and binds up their wounds"* (*Psalm* 147:3). If we let go of our bitterness and express our hurts to Him, He performs this miracle of grace in our hearts.

> With You, Lord, is abundant grace.
> Forgive me, Lord, for my bitterness
> and heal me broken heart.
> It hurt to lose my little ones.
> But I am coming to You for healing and restoration.
> I want You, and I want to be healed.
> *"Heal me O Lord and I will be healed"*
>   *Jeremiah 17:14*

Learning Contentment

"I have learned to be content in whatever circumstances I am....in any and every circumstance I have learned the secret of being filled and going hungry, both of having abundance and suffering need."
Philippians 4:11–12

Paul, the apostle, makes it sound so easy. He learned contentment. He was able to go through life without being pushed around by what life was throwing at him. He learned through the times he went hungry, didn't have clothes, was being beaten, had a lot of provision, and was in prison. He took note of the circumstances and gained the knowledge of what it meant to go through them without his emotional state of being fluctuating with every ebb and flow. Joni Eareckson Tada writes in *When God Weeps,*

> Paul was talking about an internal quietness of heart, supernaturally given, that gladly submits to God in all circumstances. When I say "quietness of heart" I'm not ruling out the physical stuff like prison bars, wheelchairs, unjust treatment, and disease. What I am ruling out is the internal stuff—peevish thoughts, plotting ways of escape, and vexing and fretting that only lead to a flurry of frantic activity. Contentment is a sedate spirit that is able to keep quiet as it bears up under suffering. Paul understood how to live this way. (171)
>
> When it comes to contentment, God must be our aim. Whether it's wayward thoughts, bad mouthing our circumstances, or comparing ourselves with others whose lot in life is easier, the battle involves more than eschewing evil; *it involves pursuing God.* (179)

Often we think contentment is "coping with the awful" and "grudgingly enduring." But I am learning that contentment is being filled with more of God and less of the circumstances. This is not easy, and perhaps that's why we have to learn it. When we learn contentment, joy begins to seep into our hearts. It is easy to look to the future and despise the current circumstances. But it is much more satisfying to *live* in the present and hope in the LORD. I believe that this can be obtained by surrendering our expectations to the LORD. He knows our dreams and the plans He has for us (Jeremiah 29:11). We can share with Him and ask Him to teach us contentment and fulfillment.

Contentment means your heart is full and peaceful with the present time. God has given us life, and we are to live in it and enjoy it. Contentment is being full of the LORD. We can feast on Him and become content. Like a good meal, we will not hunger for anything else when we "taste and see that He is good." Jesus says, "I am the bread of life; he who comes to Me will not hunger, and he who believes in Me will never thirst" (John 6:35). This is a promise of contentment in Him. "If anyone is thirsty, let him come to Me and drink. He who believes in Me, as the scripture said, from his innermost being will flow rivers of living water" (John 7:37–38). He is the fountain we can come to drink from when we are thirsty and not content (Psalm 36:9, Jeremiah 2:13, Isaiah 55:1–2).

> The psalmist writes,
> Whom have I in heaven but You? And besides You, I desire nothing on earth. My flesh and my heart may fail, but God is the strength of my heart and my portion forever. For, behold those who are far from you will perish…But as for me, the nearness of God is my good.
>
> Psalm 73:25–28.

The psalmist is truly satisfied with the nearness of God and is running to Him to be filled.

If it seems out of reach to be content, the good news is that it is found in a person and not in right circumstances or any other earthly thing. We can come to Him and ask (John 4:10).

> Lord, teach me to be content.
> Grant me grace to come and drink from You.
> I'm thirsty…
> Fill me up with living water and more of You.
> Give me grace to quietly surrender and bear up under these circumstances.
> Help me to see what You have blessed me with and not what I have not.
> Teach me to delight in You.

Thank You for bringing me contentment.
"'My people will be satisfied with My goodness,'
declares the Lord."

Jeremiah 31:14

The Father Runs to You

"So he got up and went to his father. But while He was
still a long way off, his father saw him and was filled
with compassion for him; he ran to his son, threw his
arms around him and kissed him."

Luke 15:20

I must have read the Luke 15 passage of the prodigal son many times before being enlightened by my
former professor, Pastor Phil McCallum. He lectured
about the love of the Father shown in the parable.
This passage isn't only about the prodigal son but
about the character of the Father. There in this story
is God's heart for us. A Father that runs to the son!
What a concept!

What is amazing about this passage is that even
more than our own attempts to run to God, He is
running to us. He is looking for us like a lady's precious heirloom and a shepherd's lost sheep. God is
not standing looking at us and shaking His head in
disappointment; He isn't in denial of our condition.

He is looking and watching the horizon for us to come. Then when we are still a long way off, He runs to us and embraces us.

God's promise to us is that as we draw near to Him, He will draw near to us (James 4:8). He isn't far from us (Acts 17:27). He is like the Father who runs to his son, in his time of need. I pray this would bring healing to your heart as you ponder His love for you.

Thank you, Father, for Your love that brings forgiveness with open arms. It's Your love that embraces us while we are still far off. Please teach me about Your character and this love. As much as I desire to run to You, I need You to run to me.

Comforter

"But I tell you the truth, it is to your advantage that I go away; For if I do not go away, the Helper [Paracletos, one called alongside to help, Comforter, Advocate, Intercessor] will not come to you; but if I go I will send Him to you."
John 16:7

Jesus promised His departure was to the disciples' advantage because it meant He would send a Helper and Comforter—the Holy Spirit. This may have seemed puzzling to them at the time. They were already having a hard time with the death and resurrection that Jesus told them would occur. But here was another promise, one that He said made it worth it. "*It is to your advantage,*" He says.

It is hard to fathom this "advantage" until you experience intense suffering. It is in suffering and pain that we find the One who is our Help and Comfort. He is the One who walks alongside and carries the burden, who weeps with you, who stands by you, and who wipes every tear from your eye.

It was a promised advantage. He would be with you forever (John 14:16).

Many New Testament disciples experienced God's comfort as a result of the Holy Spirit. In intense pain Stephen, "being full of the Holy Spirit," was able to "fall asleep" as he was being stoned (Acts 7:55, 60). Paul was experiencing persecution, and "the LORD stood at his side" and encouraged him (Acts 23:11). He knew the One who comes alongside. The early church experienced the Comforter, "So the church throughout all Judea and Galilee and Samaria enjoyed peace, being built up; and going on in the fear of the LORD and *in the comfort of the Holy Spirit,* it continued to increase" (Acts 9:31).

When we run to Him, we find that He is waiting and ready to comfort and help us in our time of need. "Therefore let us draw near with confidence to the throne of grace, so that we may receive mercy and find grace to help in time of need" (Hebrews 4:16).

The Comfort He Brings

> Blessed be the God and Father of our LORD Jesus Christ, the Father of mercies and God of all comfort, who comforts us in all our affliction so that we will be able to comfort those who are in any affliction with the comfort with which we ourselves are comforted by God. For just as the sufferings of Christ are ours in abundance, so also our comfort is abundant through Christ.
>
> 2 Corinthians 1:3–5

The God of all comfort promises to comfort us in all afflictions. This is a pretty hefty promise. It can be challenge to believe this promise is even true. It may seem hard to believe because it is not easy to see the comfort. The pain of the suffering may blind us to the comfort of a friend, a kind word, a hug, or a warm embrace. We may miss the very messenger God is sending to bring the comfort our souls need. We may overlook a card, some flowers, or just a friendly gesture.

God chooses to let us experience Him as Comforter, *and* He also chooses to use frail people to show His love and comfort. And through the process He uses our hurts to comfort others. When we get hurt, He comforts us, people comfort us, and in turn, we comfort others. The very truth that your suffering is not in vain and it indeed will be used to comfort others can bring healing to your heart. God doesn't waste a hurt. He fills us up with comfort and transforms us into people who are able to show compassion. We are then ready to weep with those who weep (Romans 12:15).

"'Comfort, O Comfort My people,' says your God."
Isaiah 40:1

Oh Lord, I am so grateful for Your Comfort and the healing You bring. Thank You that You are the Comforter, Holy Spirit. Please heal and comfort my heart. Help me understand suffering and make me more like You, that I could bring comfort to others as they suffer.

Understanding Suffering

"For if He causes grief, then He will have compassion according to His abundant lovingkindness for He does not afflict willingly. Or grieve the sons of men."
Lamentations 3:32–33

As my heart began to receive His comfort, and I experienced suffering, it stirred in me a desire to understand better what suffering was. Why was I going through it? How could God bring me comfort and yet allow the affliction?

Was it a package deal? Hosea talks about a call for Israel to return to the LORD, *"For He has torn us, but He will heal us; He has wounded us, but He will bandage us"* (*Hosea* 6:1). It didn't make sense to me. I was being comforted and healed. Was the same hand that hurt me healing me?

It can be very difficult to make sense of suffering. This next chapter is devoted to exploring suffering.

Lessons from Paul

"For you it has been granted for Christ's sake, not only to believe in Him, but also to suffer for His sake, experiencing the same conflict which you saw in me, and now hear to be in me."

Phil. 1:29–30

Paul writes this to the church at Philippi (Phil. 1:29–30). The apostle Paul knew suffering. From his very first encounter with Christ he was blinded. His conversion was not simply a hand gesture or a joyful kneeling. He became blind. Ananias was sent to him with these words, "Go for he is a chosen instrument of Mine, to bear My name before the Gentiles and kings and the sons of Israel; *for I will show him how much he must suffer for My name's sake*" (*Acts* 9:15–16). Paul writes about his experience in his letters to the Corinthian church, "Five times I received from the Jews thirty-nine lashes. Three times I was beaten with rods, once I was stoned, three times I was shipwrecked, a night and a day I have spent in the deep" (2 Corinthians 11:24–25). When I read about Paul, I think, "What kind of Christianity is that?" Supposedly, it is the same. But somehow suffering is not in the current "Christianese" vocabulary.

Now I have heard many different views on suffering, but it is a rare topic of the pulpit. I have read about the apostles and their persecution, but why is that when suffering occurs in my life and in the world around me, I am shocked and often dismayed? Paul seems to handle it well.

Often I think someone or something is at fault for the suffering that takes place on a day-to-day basis. Who is behind it all? Is it God, sin, or the enemy? Perhaps it is circumstantial? Perhaps it is consequential? Perhaps it is deeper than all of this?

In my experience, suffering comes with a package deal that is puzzling. In its wrapping, I have found grief, mourning, loss, pain, emotional distress, and anger.

Suffering and Anger

I have experienced a lot of anger over the loss of my babies as well as others whom I have prayed for. At times, the anger seemed to be misdirected like an aimless ping pong ball; anger at God, anger at myself, anger at sin, suffering, and even the devil himself. Behind the anger is a little girl deep inside who has been hurt. What seems to be most frustrating in these circumstances is that there is nothing you can do. You can only feel it. It rises up inside of you demanding that you act out on it. Ironically, it is easy to be angry at your own anger.

"Be angry, and yet do not sin; do not let the sun go down on your own anger" (Ephesians 4:26). Anger, according to Paul, seems to be a natural human response, but it needs to be controlled. The Psalmist David offers some counsel, "Tremble with anger or fear, and do not sin; meditate in your heart upon your bed, and be still" (Psalm 4:4).

At times, I feel as though I had been shot in the heart and a chasm remains. I see it and I hurt. But angrily I cannot fix myself. What can I do? I can pray and I can be comforted by God's Word. But when this anger aches inside of you all you really feel like doing is escaping. You feel as though the last thing you want to do is run to God. This is such a mystery because deep down in our souls we know that He is the only one that can really help.

Lord, I pray that somehow You would soften my heart and help me to run to You. I ask that You take my anger and turn it into compassion for the suffering. I ask that You would comfort me and help me to open up to Your comfort. Please Lord, grant me self control over my anger by the power of Your Spirit. Please encourage me with the hope of being with You forever, let that be my gain as I take up my cross. Amen.

Suffering as the Unwanted Mystery

Suffering is an enigma. We all will experience loss, persecution, illness, tragic accidents, and devastation. This seems to be the biggest unwanted mystery no one has found an answer to. There are lots of mysteries out there, and we spend lots of time trying to understand why they are so. But when it comes to suffering, I do not think we have made any headway. Perhaps it is one of those mysteries that we will never fully understand until we stand before God. If so, we still remain in pain for the lack of resolution to our sufferings. There seem to be many facets and factors in what we think causes suffering, but we all agree that it exists.

People have attributed the cause of suffering to: sinful people, a fallen world, personal consequences, the devil, by chance, natural disasters, and even God. The following is an excerpt that my husband wrote on suffering.

Understanding God and Suffering

The emergency room is cold and lonely as our tears fall. Sobs that refuse to be comforted sink into the clean, sanitary walls. I weep with my wife over our second lost child—leaving the world before even being born. What is this thing called suffering, and why does it happen? More importantly, why does it happen to me?—or not to me? (as survivors of the World Trade Center are asking). Where does tragedy come from? And most importantly, where is God in all of this? In the next few pages, we will take an in-depth look at what the Bible has to say about suffering and how Christians should respond to tragedy.

What Is Suffering?

When we hear the word *suffering* we think of pain, death, anguish, etc. Starving people suffer. Prisoners suffer. Slaves suffer. Suffering is something we are all likely to endure in some form and something we work daily to avoid. The first thing to notice about suffering is that it is as inescapable as sin—and that, perhaps, gives us a clue to its source. The Bible tells us that suffering is not part of God's original creation or plan for humanity. This is clear from a short examination of texts relating to pre-fall creation. First, we see that suffering is *introduced* to Adam and Eve *after* they sinned in Genesis 3:16–19,

> To the woman He said, "I will greatly multiply Your pain in childbirth, In pain you shall bring forth children; Yet your desire shall be for your husband, And he shall rule over you."
>
> Then to Adam He said, "...Cursed is the ground because of you; In toil you shall eat of it All the days of your life.
> Both thorns and thistles it shall grow for you; And you shall eat the plants of the field; By the sweat of your face You shall eat bread, Till you return to the ground..."

The most glaring thing here is the implication that childbirth, one of the most painful things known to man, was intended to be considerably less painful. Also, the suffering of difficult work to get food was introduced here implying that sustaining a living from the land was intended to be much easier. Lastly, along this line we see in Revelation 7:17 that when God restores all things our struggle against suffering will be over, "The Lamb...shall be their shepherd, and shall guide them to springs of the water of life; and God shall *wipe* every *tear* from their eyes."

Why Does Suffering Happen?

In our quest to avoid suffering, or to at least understand it when it comes, we must grapple with the question "What causes suffering?" While the Bible does imply one single *origin* of suffering, the entry of sin into the world, it does not declare just one immediate *cause* of suffering. By looking at many passages on suffering, I have found it helpful to group the circumstances of suffering into three broad categories: 1) Suffering by Chance, 2) Suffering by Law, 3) Suffering by Design.

Suffering by chance is derived from observing events which can only be explained in terms of coincidence. It is based mainly on two important doctrines. First, the doctrine that *God does not usually interfere with the laws of time and space* as we know them. The miracle of Jesus walking on water (Mark 6:45ff), the parting of the Red Sea (Exodus 14:13ff), and Phillip's transportation (Acts 8:39–40) are exceptions that prove this rule. In most situations, God does not do these kinds of miraculous things—they are miraculous specifically because they are not the norm. The second doctrine is the doctrine of *free will.* Without a lengthy debate on this issue, we will take it for granted here that, biblically speaking, God usually does not make decisions for people—people make decisions themselves.

The conclusion we can draw from these two doctrines is that coincidences, good and bad, are both possible and to be expected in everyday life. Suffering can, in fact, happen because a person literally puts himself in the wrong place at the wrong time. The writer of Ecclesiastes comments, "I again saw under the sun that the race is not to the swift, and the battle is not to the warriors, and neither is bread to the wise, nor wealth to the discerning, nor favor to men of ability; *for time and chance* overtake them all" (Ecc. 9:11). This does not mean that God is not sovereign or not ultimately in control, but rather that "God's sovereignty...transcends human freedom but does not nullify it. Both are real..." (Sittser, 142).

Suffering by Law is the straightforward doctrine that "whatever a man sows, this he will also reap" (Gal. 6:7) and "those who plow iniquity [or] those who sow trouble harvest it" (Job 4:8). The law of sowing and reaping is one of the basic laws of the Bible. If a person violates God's law, whether that law is written on stone tablets or a law "written in their hearts" (Rom. 2:15), consequences of retribution will follow—usually causing suffering. I am not talking about suffering personally inflicted by God to punish sinners here, but rather suffering that comes about as a natural consequence to sin. Although this one is "a given," I'd like to point out that, in almost every case of suffering by law, the cause of suffering will be obvious. Either a person's own conscience will condemn him, or God Himself will send a clear rebuke and conviction. If you are laboring under a nebulous cloud of oppressive condemnation because you think your suffering is *suffering by law,* only you don't know which law you have broken, and no clear conviction is arising, rebuke the condemnation!—it is clearly from Satan. This is something I have had to deal with regarding the miscarriage because Satan wants me to think I did something wrong which caused it, and to kill myself in condemning over-examination trying to find out what my sin was. Tricky, isn't he?

Suffering by design can be understood when we consider Job's plight in the Bible. We can see that Job's accusing friends thought he was *suffering by law,* but Job knew he had broken no law! Chapter after agonizing chapter, Job's friends try to convince him that he must've offended God somehow, and Job tries to convince them that God is making him suffer *by design.* Job is a man totally destroyed by suffering, and he is naturally genuinely mad at God for allowing or sending these hardships. Job accuses God of being unfair and even borders on accusing God of being evil rather than good, "Thou hast become *cruel*

to me; With the might of Thy hand Thou dost persecute me" (Job 30:21).

God reacts to Job in two ways which support Job's
belief that he is suffering *by design*. First, He rebukes
Job for his prideful insolence in accusing God, "Will
the faultfinder contend with the Almighty? Let him
who reproves God answer it" (Job 40:2). God is, in
effect, saying, "Yes, you are suffering by my design but
who are you to accuse me of being cruel?" Secondly,
God rebukes Job's friends saying, "My wrath is kin-
dled against you…because you have not spoken of Me
what is right as My servant Job has" (Job 42:7). The
main thing Job spoke about God could be summarized like this, "God is the Ultimate, Sovereign Being
in the universe, and He does whatever He wants—He
is right now choosing to crush me for no apparent
reason." The main thing Job's friends argued could
be summarized as, "Justice is a universal principle by
which even God abides, and so you must be suffering
because you have sinned." From these observations,
we can see that Job's friends failed to understand the
sovereignty of God and so did not understand *suffering by design*.

There are many examples in the Bible of *suffering
by* design, including the times in the Bible where *God
is inflicting* judgment on sinful people or nations. For
instance, God personally enforces the consequences
for the sin of Korah in the Old Testament, "But if

the LORD brings about an entirely new thing and the ground opens its mouth and swallows them up with all that is theirs, and they descend alive into Sheol, then you will understand that these men have spurned the LORD" (Num. 16:29). In the New Testament, this is seen when God strikes Ananias and Sapphira dead for trying to deceive the church and the LORD. In addition, suffering is often *designed and inflicted by Satan,* as in the story of Job, the stoning of Stephen, or the persecution of the early Christian church. Jesus said to Peter, "Simon, Simon, behold, Satan has demanded *permission* to sift you like wheat..." (Luke 22:31).

Through these examples, we can see that much of suffering is *by design,* through God's direct action or permission—but that *does not include all suffering.* We can also suffer by *law,* or by *chance.* So, in answer to the question "Why does suffering happen?" we can see several clear answers:

- Suffering happens by chance because of freewill and natural law,
- Suffering happens as a consequence of law breaking and sin,
- Suffering happens by God's design or permission.

In most cases, suffering is the result of a combination of these causes.

Why God?

All of us will ask the question, *"Why God?"* when we experience either suffering by chance or suffering by design. In the case of suffering by chance, we are really asking, "God, *why didn't You* intervene to stop this?" Sometimes the answer is that the person suffering could not hear God warn him, perhaps because that person did not have a relationship with God. Such is the case of Paul's shipwreck in Acts 27. Paul "perceive[s] that the voyage will certainly be attended with damage and great loss," but "the centurion was more persuaded by the pilot and the captain of the ship than by…Paul" (Acts 27:10–11). Sometimes there is no satisfactory answer, except that a fallen world, bound by laws of space and time and full of sinful self-directing human beings, is certain to cause tragic suffering—and this is *not how God originally designed the world to be.*

"Now wait a minute!" you say. "I'm tired of all this talk about chance. There are no 'chances'; God has a purpose for everything!" I know where you're coming from, and you're right, God does have a purpose for everything. But let's look back at the shipwreck. It is clear that God *transformed* the shipwreck into great ministry opportunities for Paul, but it is also clear that the *cause* of the shipwreck was the foolish choices made by the captain, pilot, and centurion. Even though God knew about this from the beginning of time, He did not motivate or inflict it—but He did *redeem* it! God is so intensely creative and powerful that He can redeem any situation. In this way, God has a purpose for everything, but that doesn't mean He *causes* everything.

When we suffer by design, what we're really asking is "God, *why did You* do this to me?" Job asked this question. So did Joseph, David, Jesus' disciples, and many others. In hindsight, we can see that the answer is always the same, *redemptive transformation*. Job, at the end of his suffering, was proved righteous, blessed even more abundantly, and was able to say, "I had heard about you [God] before, but now I have seen you with my own eyes" (Job 42:5). Joseph became a great man of God and saved the known world from starvation, including his family. David became perhaps the most humble king there has ever been, after he spent years hiding in caves from Saul. And Jesus...

Where Is God in All of This?

As Christians, we have a unique perspective on suffering. For us the central figure in human history is Jesus Christ, "a man of sorrows and aquatinted with grief" (Is. 53:3) and the central event in human history is His crucifixion on a Roman cross for the sins of the world. Through Jesus' suffering, all people who suffer can know that God is near to them; that God *experientially understands* how they feel. Jesus suffered as deeply as anyone has ever suffered, and Jesus' death was the greatest tragedy of all tragedies and also the greatest victory of all victories.

Where is God in our sufferings? In the middle, smack dab in the middle. Jesus came to earth and suffered terribly so that no one could ever again say, "God is far away from me and doesn't understand how I feel." All people who experience suffering find that this truth comforts their souls deeply. I believe that God has suffered more than anyone will ever suffer since He has suffered with everyone who has ever suffered. If we are suffering by chance, where is He? He is standing by, hearing our prayers, and working redemptive miracles from terrible circumstances like Paul's shipwreck. If we are suffering by law, where is He? He is dying on a cross under the weight of God's punishment for that sin, so we wouldn't have to bear it. If we are suffering by design, where is He? He is by our side, carrying the heavy-end of the yoke, and doing everything He can to work a redemptive transformation in us. Through God's acts in history, especially the incarnation, we can know for certain that when we are suffering, God is there!

How Should We Respond?

When we talk about Jesus' death, we must view it as inseparable from his life before and resurrection after the event. From our vantage point in history, we can see the tremendous triumph of the cross. We can see the incredible transformation, which the cross makes possible in the lives of individuals. To our eyes, the cross of Christ is a transformational victory. But that's not how Jesus' disciples saw it. All they could see was a terrible tragedy. When Jesus was taken prisoner, they were thrown into confusion. Most ran away. Peter followed but denied he even knew Jesus. After His death, they were holed up in a room where "the doors were shut…for fear of the Jews…" (John 20:19). They would have stayed this way indefinitely had not the LORD appeared to them, talked with them, ate with them, and convinced them that He was risen. Then, for the rest of their lives, they grew more and more in understanding how the suffering of Jesus and the tragedy of His death had a wonderful purpose!

All of us in the midst of tragedy react as Jesus' disciples did: in confusion, in fear, in disbelief, in shock, in depression, in anger, and in all other kinds of despondency. We can hardly be expected to act otherwise—after all, Jesus did not expect more of His disciples but told them plainly, "You will all fall away, because it is written, '*I will strike down the shepherd, and the sheep shall be scattered*'" (Mark 14:27). The disciples had the privilege of being told directly by the LORD that there was a purpose to His suffering and a great hope: the resurrection. Nevertheless, they lost all hope until the LORD revealed His risen self to them.

When we suffer, we are no different than the disciples. We too have been promised a resurrection to eternal life. We have been promised "that God causes *all things* to work together *for good* to those who love God, to those who are called according to *His* purpose" (Romans 8:28). Though we can't see it now, there will be a day in which everything is set right, and on that glorious day God Himself will "…*wipe away every tear* from [our] eyes; and there shall no longer be *any* death; there shall no longer be *any* mourning, or crying, or pain…" (Rev. 21:4). We believe deep in our hearts that on that day all the pain and suffering will finally make sense, and we will clearly see God's wonderful, transformational, purpose. That is our great hope. Yet from this day, where we stand knee-deep in suffering, we can hardly see that hope at all.

What shall we do then? Let us not grow stoic or surreal and pretend not to feel, and try to look like stalwart, strong, hopeful people. For many of us, a reaction like that would be a lie. Let us instead be true to ourselves as the disciples were—confused, afraid, questioning, disbelieving—and deeply longing still for our savior in what feels like a hopeless situation. Let us trust Jesus to come to us in the midst of our trial and, with His good shepherd's hands, carry us not away from suffering, but through it. Let us ask Him plainly the questions in our minds and trust that His answer, though maybe not the one we were hoping for, will satisfy our souls. Most of all, let us run hard or trudge or crawl or fall *toward* our Savior and never away.

–Koa Siu

Why Not Me?

At some point in my journey of processing suffering and the loss we experienced, I stumbled upon a question, "Why not me?" I have to admit that I did ask the inevitable "why me" question. But there came a moment where I sat back and thought, Really...why not me? Who am I that I should never suffer? It's silly when I think about it. I'm not immune to pain. Some kind of unrealistic self-righteous attitude was hanging over me. What was I thinking? Was I always expecting to be the one to "win the lottery" and get the blessings of God while not accepting the much more common "better luck next time" ticket?

Job accepted both. His wife's response to the loss and tragedy they experienced was for Job to "curse God and die!" While Job says, *"You speak as one of the foolish women speaks. Shall we indeed accept good from God and not accept adversity?"* (Job 2:9–10).

Something in me needed to learn and mature. I am not one to dwell on martyrdom. I don't think I have that gift. But I began to realize the One I am following was acquainted with sorrows and walked to the cross. He says I can expect trials and persecution, *"If they persecuted Me, they will also persecute you"* (John 15:20). Somehow that had dropped off the radar of my life. Perhaps if I lived in a place hostile to the gospel, I might know firsthand about such suffering. I had such a great conversion. He saved me from so much sin and suffering. The life I lived in Christ seemed, like Job's, to be filled with blessings. My childlike faith believed if I prayed for these babies to live, they would!

I needed to know that God did want to bless me, but He also wants me to follow Him, even if that

means going through dark times and places. I needed
a new commitment to Him that I would follow Him
even if it meant walking through the valley of the
shadow of death. The good news about walking there
is that He is with me there too. Here are some promises that He is there in the dark times and places:

> Even though I walk through the valley of the
> shadow of death, I fear no evil, for You are with
> me; Your rod and Your staff, they comfort me.
>
> Psalm 23:4

> If I ascend to heaven, You are there; If I make
> my bed in Sheol, behold, You are there. If
> I take the wings of the dawn, if I dwell in
> the remotest part of the sea, even there Your
> hand will lead me, and Your right hand will
> lay hold of me. If I say, "Surely the darkness
> will overwhelm me, and the light around me
> will be night," even the darkness is not dark
> to You, and the night is as bright as the day.
> Darkness and light are alike to You.
>
> Psalm 139:8–12

I had to ask myself some tough questions. Not
to mention feeling as though God Himself was asking me, "Is it enough for you to become like your

Master?" This struck my heart. "It is enough for the disciple that he become like his teacher, and the slave like his master?" (Matthew 10:25).

About a year after our first miscarriage, my husband and I went to a missions conference. During the worship one night, I felt the presence of the LORD very strongly and heard, "Can you drink the cup I drink?" I started crying and sat down, and I was speechless. I didn't know how to answer. But I knew the passage.

James and John wanted Jesus to do whatever they asked Him to do (Mark 10:35). They wanted to sit with Him in His glory. Jesus responded, "You do not know what you are asking. Are you able to drink the cup that I drink or to be baptized with the baptism with which I am baptized?" They said yes! They would too! I wonder if they ever felt like they had stuck their foot in their mouth.

I spent three months contemplating this question that I heard at the conference. In one of my old journals, I asked Him what He meant. I felt an impression that the cup was His cross. Jesus says in the Garden of Gethsemane, "Abba, Father! All things are possible for You; *remove this cup from Me;* yet not what I will, but what You will" (Mark 14:36). He was asking me to suffer as He had. Could I take up my cross and follow? Could I drink the same cup? Would I?

I would embrace it. I did. I do. I will. Why not

me? What better person to handle suffering than a follower of Jesus? Someone He could use to touch others and comfort them in their time of need. Someone whom He could redeem the hurts and mold more into His image.

Oh Lord, thank You for choosing me. I realize that I am following You. And sometimes You walk through dark places. Help me to drink the cup of Your cross that I might walk with You every day and everywhere.

"And when He had taken a cup and given thanks, He gave it to them, and they all drank from it." (Mark 14:23)

Conformed to His Image

"And we know that God causes all things to work together for good to those who love God, to those who are called according to His purpose. For those whom He foreknew, He also pre-destined to become conformed to the image of His Son…"
Romans 8:28–29

On a few occasions, I experienced the above scripture at a trite cliché thrown at me like it was coming from left field. "God was going to work it all out for the good," I'd hear. When you're going through loss, it does not seem to apply to the pain you are feeling nor have a landing place in a hurting heart because it is just too hard to see the "good" in tragedy. What good is there in the loss of a child or in the death of lots of innocent people?

This scripture and promise has a time in each person's life. Some may find the good; some may not. Perhaps the simple truth is that God will continue to take what isn't good and redeem it for His purposes, which are good. God can take the loss and a person in pain suffering the loss and infuse purpose into it.

But His ultimate purpose according to this scripture is to conform us into the image of His Son. Being conformed to His image is a byproduct of suffering. It is a high calling to become more like Him (Romans 8:30). The suffering we undergo conforms us into His image.

What's He Like?

"He was despised and forsaken of men, a man of sorrows and acquainted with grief...surely our grief He Himself bore, and our sorrows He carried"
Isaiah 53:3–4

You may be asking yourself, "Do I really want to be conformed into the image of someone well acquainted with sorrows?" In this day and age, it may seem more appealing to want to be a movie star, or someone with earthly success, an "easy" life, and all the bells and whistles to go with it. Do I really want to be conformed into the image of Jesus? Well, to answer this question, it's pertinent to explore who He is and what He is like.

In her book *When God Weeps,* Joni Eareckson Tada, explains, "Take this reverently; snap a photo of Jesus and you've got God on film" (36). Jesus said, "I and the Father are One" (John 10:30). "He is the image of the invisible God" (Colossians 1:15). We can see what God is like because of Jesus.

Jesus' life and ministry were painted with beautiful moments of compassion, love, healing after healing, miracles of provision, and devotion to do God's will. He had compassion on the crowds as well as individuals. "*Seeing the people, He felt compassion for them, because they were distressed and dispirited like sheep without a shepherd*" (*Matthew* 9:36).

He deeply cared for others and was accepting of lepers, outcasts, prostitutes, and the "untouchables" of His time. His tenderness spilled over for children as well. His love is undefeatable.

Perhaps what I admire most about Him is that He overcomes. He does the Father's will despite suffering or pain that is before Him.

I don't like to clean the refrigerator. In fact, I detest it. I abhor it most when there is some unknown substance that takes on the form of superglue and causes drawers to be unavailable for anyone to use. One afternoon, I was fed up. I was going to attack the sticky mess. I had to psyche myself up and prepare. To my surprise, the amount of wiping and Clorox had no affect on the mysterious sludge. I had to let it sit. And inside I thought, *I need help*. I could barely reach in there and get it, not to mention my scrubbing was not successful.

I sprayed it with more Clorox and waited. I waited until my husband came home. I was going to ask him for help. He was so gracious and said something along the lines of "my pleasure." He cheerfully and easily wiped it down, and it was like it had been no big deal. Granted there were reasons for his success, like the soaking of a highly potent chemical for several hours. But he overcame it.

It is noteworthy that he did it with a good heart and, despite getting on his hands and knees, with the full knowledge that it might be really hard to scrub off. He did it.

Jesus was willing to go to the darkest, hardest limits for love. He had the full knowledge of what it meant to go to the cross. He overcame betrayal, loss, and death itself. He didn't let anything stop Him from doing the Father's will. He did for you and me.

I don't know about you, but that is something I really need to be conformed to. I would pass on tests, trials, and suffering all together if I had my option.

Perhaps that's why He uses sufferings and trials to strengthen my resolve. I surely need to be conformed into His image.

Test of Faith

> "In this you greatly rejoice, even though now for a little while, if necessary, you have been distressed by various trials, so that the proof of your faith, being more precious than gold which is perishable, even though tested by fire, may be found to result in praise and glory and honor at the revelation of Jesus Christ,"
>
> 1 Peter 1:6–7

Imagine it's finals week. For some this may be hard to picture, having been out of school for quite some time. But picture it; you are entering a time of extreme testing. It's time to review notes, re-read books, or read them for the first time! It's time to memorize and make sure the knowledge that has been spewed out before you, has been digested. It's a time for anxiety, uncertainty, and prayer! You might pray that the exam would be canceled, postponed, or simply that it would be easy. If you are like me, you may be thinking, "What are these tests good for?"

In life, we are faced with "tests" or "trials." The

challenges life throws at us are often a lot harder than an exam. These often leave us feeling shaken up inside.

In these trials, the proof of your faith may be found. They prove what you really believe. You see, much like a final exam, tests reveal what you *really* know. When you take the test, what is really inside of you is what you pass with. It's the things you understand that come up from within you when you are tested. These things that you understand will shine forth.

But the things you only know in part will also show. Things that you just memorized in your head will not. Wrong answers will also surface and things you did not take seriously.

So tests distinguish between what's in your head and what's in your heart.

On a personal level, I can remember a time when I was tested on what I said I know and what I committed to walk out. Before I met my husband, Koa, I committed myself not to have a boyfriend until I knew that I would marry him. I decided to give up dating. Well, as I started to get more serious about it, I was tested three times to see if I would really trust God. This trial proved that this conviction was in me that my faith was real I really wanted to walk with the LORD in this area. The trial brought out my faith in God, to carry me through and trust that He really had someone out there for me. It revealed my heart and what I really knew as true. At the same time, it showed me what I still needed to work on.

You might be thinking, "Why is this important?" Well, because this faith we have saves us. "It is by grace that you have been saved through faith; and that not of yourselves, it is a gift of God" (Ephesians 2:8). It also results in glory, love, and honor to Jesus. This is the real stuff! This refined faith causes us to "love Him, though we don't see Him, we greatly rejoice, with joy inexpressible and full of glory, obtaining as the outcome of our faith the salvation of your souls" (1 Peter 1:8–9).

The one thing we can have in this world is our faith, belief, and trust in Jesus. It's the one eternal thing worth value in our life. Without this, there is no meaning to life. Your faith in Jesus is the one thing that sets you apart from the rest of the world.

Nothing could be more precious. It is the pearl that the merchant sold everything for (Matt. 13:45). This faith that is being refined is priceless. It's more precious than gold.

It's worth all the trials you could go through!

Trials are also good because they bring about perseverance, proven character, and hope. Romans 5:3–5 says,

> And not only this but we also exult in tribulations, knowing that tribulations brings about perseverance; and perseverance, proven charac-

ter; and proven character, hope; and hope does not disappoint, because the love of God has been poured out within our hearts through the Holy Spirit who was given to us.

Trials push us to a point where we need to decide to keep going or give up. Suffering stretches our character to choose to persevere with the LORD.

When things get tough, we will either push through or sit on the sideline. And even if we push through, there is a possibility we will do it begrudgingly. My actions may say, "yes," but my attitude says, "no." Through the process, our character is "proven." When you're in a jam, how do you respond? This is pretty straightforward. When you are in traffic, do you get frustrated and let out a sigh or groan?

I remember a certain year when we had our taxes done. Unfortunately, the person who did our taxes did not file our taxes correctly. She did not include half of my income. Now this was a trial, and to make matters worse, we picked them up from her three hours before the deadline! The way I responded revealed a lot about my character. I was frustrated and was working through forgiving her because we needed to redo everything. I could tell I needed to have more grace and patience. My character needed work. I learned a lot about my character from how I responded to the whole situation.

Trials also bring hope. Through trials, we learn

how to put our trust in the LORD. We learn to look to Him to sustain us, to deliver us, and to fulfill His promises. We learn to hope in Him and not just for the situation to get better.

Trials are good because they bring us closer to God through repentance. "For the sorrow that is according to the will of God produces a repentance without regret, leading to salvation" (2 Corinthians 7:9–10). Paul writes that sorrow can lead you to repentance. Repentance is basically turning to the LORD. I like to define it as choosing to draw near to God. Trials that sometimes seem so painful lead us to our knees. Trials bring us to a place where we can run to the Father just as Jesus did in the Garden of Gethsemane. He was filled with sorrow at the test He was about to face. It drove Him to the Father, much like we are driven to the Father. *Trials give you the opportunity to run to the Lord, to run to His presence.*

Once we get into His embrace, it may not all make sense, but it is the best place to be.

Learning from Peter

"Simon, son of John, do you love Me?"
John 21:16

One of the most powerful lessons I have learned from the Apostle Simon Peter's life is *not to base my faith on my own expectations.* I realized that prior to my first miscarriage, suffering was not part of my Christian vocabulary. My faith was based on the underlying assumptions of who and what "I" thought God to be like. Sometimes our assumptions can be distorted and different from the Word of God. Like Peter, I probably would have rebuked the LORD for His announcement of the cross. The story is told in Mark 8:27–38. Jesus asks the disciples, "Who do people say that I am?"

They responded, "John the Baptist; and others say Elijah; but others, one of the prophets."

Then Jesus probed further, "But who do you say that I am?"

Peter answered, "You are the Christ." I wonder how he said it. I wonder if it was like an eager student, reciting everyone else's wrong answer. "I know! I know!" earnestly raising his hand. Or I wonder if he solemnly contemplated the discussion by process of elimination, "Well He's not John and He's not Elijah..."

In the book of Matthew, we see that it was not flesh and blood that revealed this to Peter, but the Father in heaven (16:17). Peter knew He was the Messiah because the Father had revealed it to him. What was not revealed to Peter was that Jesus would have to suffer for the sins of the world. Peter may have expected the Messiah to build His kingdom here on earth and overthrow the oppressive government of that time.

"And He began to teach them that the Son of Man must suffer many things and be rejected by the elders the chief priests and the scribes, and be killed, and after three days rise again" (Mark 8:31). Hmm, that can't be right Jesus. That doesn't make sense. "He was stating the matter plainly. And Peter took Him aside and began to rebuke Him" (vs. 32). I wonder what Peter said. Did he argue that that was not what the Messiah was to do? "But turning around and seeing His disciples, He rebuked Peter and said, 'Get behind me Satan; for you are not setting your mind on God's interests, but man's'" (vs. 33).

Here Jesus told them plainly that He was going to suffer and die. This was shocking to them. I think it is still shocking to me. Our society opposes suffering and strives at every attempt to relieve it. Like Job's friends, we accuse those who suffer to be in sin. Thinking that righteousness is living a comfortable, healthy, and perfect life. We are taught from an early age that suffering is not right. Perhaps this is because it involves so much pain and emotion. Well, I am not saying we should enjoy it or go out looking for suffering, but we should not deny that people suffer. As long as we are here on earth we will have heartache. I am also not saying that He does not heal or want us to be healed. Simply, I am saying that if our own expectations push us to blame Jesus and "rebuke" him like Peter, there is something else going on. Why is it that when we get hurt we are so quick to blame God? Why is it that when we suffer we think He is being unfair? Perhaps we have fallen prey to our own expectations about who God is and suffering.

Peter learned when faced with the cross that his faith needed to be based on Christ Himself and not on his own expectations. At the cross, Peter wept bitterly and experienced personal suffering and anguish. Then when you read on in the New Testament, Peter is a leader in the church, and he learns to put his faith in God. He preaches to the Gentiles and undergoes physical suffering. He is persecuted and imprisoned. He writes to the persecuted church,

> Beloved, do not be surprised at the fiery ordeal among you, which comes upon you for your testing, as though some strange thing were happening to you; but to the degree that you share in the sufferings of Christ, keep on

> rejoicing, so that also at the revelation of His
> glory you may rejoice with exultation....but if
> anyone suffers as a Christian, he is not to be
> ashamed, but is to glorify God in this name.
>
> 1 Peter 5:12,13,16

Somewhere down the line, Peter learned about suffering. I would say it was at the cross.

Peter's faith had to switch from being founded on his own expectation of what God would do and it needed to be faith in whom He is. Then he would truly live as the "rock" God made him to be.

Beth Moore sums it up in *Living Beyond Yourself,*

> "Do you ever tire of riding the roller coaster
> of faith? Of being up one day and down the
> next? Of believing Him one minute and not
> the next? We can exercise our faith in God
> in one of two ways. One leaves us at the
> mercy of life's roller coaster to begin walking
> with God and practicing a faith that can't be
> "greatly moved" (Ps. 61:2, KJV). Every believer
> falls into one of these two categories on the
> basis of her answer to one simple question:
> do you base your faith on what God does or
> who He is?" (163)

I have lived on the roller coaster she talks about.

There are times I still need to redirect and take a step back from the circumstances and get my faith simply in Him. I need to remind myself that He is good and whatever is going on, He remains the same.

Dear Lord, I give You my expectations. I want to have faith in You and not just what I think You should and shouldn't do. I put my faith in who You are. You are God, and You are good.

Moving Forward

Well eventually over the course of time and with God's help in healing, comes the next step. It becomes the moment where you decide to open up your heart and try once more for there to be life in your womb. This may bring up all the issues you thought you put behind you during the last miscarriage.

I found myself struggling with all sorts of mixed emotions such as *denial, unwillingness, hardness of heart,* and *defensiveness.* Yet deep in my heart, I can hear God's voice calling me to trust Him and step out in faith. Also, despite the tough front, I really knew deep down I did desire to have a child.

Denial

The first stage I found myself going through was a denial that I even wanted to have children. I had "moved on." I was doing things with my life and was not even allowing myself the luxury of dreaming about becoming pregnant. I found other things to occupy myself with and poured myself whole-heartedly into work and ministry.

It's funny how when those emotions get stirred, it can often be like a kick in the pants. I was watching *Cheaper by the Dozen,* starring Steve Martin, and although it was a funny movie, I left in tears. I realized I had closed myself off to the dream of having a family in order to pursue other things.

I felt the stirrings in my soul to be open to God, to try again, to trust that perhaps He was now finally leading me to have a child. This was different from the other two times.

God is certainly well acquainted with our "true" deep desires. He sees the inner pangs of our thirsty hearts. He isn't afraid to stir us, to "ruffle our feathers," so to speak. Much like a loving dad messes up a child's hair with a loving and assuring hand.

Scriptures portray Him as seeing the hearts of man, knowing the inner thoughts, and even answering the longings of our souls. It's hard to live in denial when there's someone who can see right through it all.

> Psalm 37:4 "Delight yourself in the LORD; And He will give you the desires of your heart."

Psalm 21:2 "You have given him his heart's desire, and You have not withheld the request of his lips."

Psalm 145:19 "He will fulfill the desire of those who fear Him; He will also hear their cry and will save them."
Mark 2:8 "Immediately Jesus, aware in His spirit that they were reasoning that way within themselves, said to them, "Why are you reasoning about these things in your hearts?"

Unwillingness

An unwillingness to try again is different from denial. With denial, a person "fools" themselves to think they really do not want what they are pursuing. Unwillingness is simply not being willing to take a risk.

For me, I felt a little unwillingness about moving forward and trying to have another baby. This feeling seems to be a response to the pain and disappointment of the previous miscarriage. There is a part of my heart that had "learned" from these experiences that I should not try, it would wise to guard my heart and spare myself the pain.

Sometimes when thinking about this, I am reminded of lab animals or small children. In some lab animals, a negative stimulus is given them in response to an action, and they adapt to not repeating the action. Or with a small child who touches something hot, the child learns not to touch it again, or else it will hurt.

But taking a look at the bigger picture helps to overcome such "learned tendencies" because, unlike a lab animal, we are called to follow Christ even if it hurts. We can find courage when we think about Christ Himself and His sacrifice. He died for us, His beloved children. This knowledge can refresh and encourage us to love past the pain and even be willing to go through the pain to try again to have another child.

He risked the pain and moved past it. In the Garden of Gethsemane, He cried out, "My Father, if it is possible, let this cup pass from Me: yet not as I, but as You will" (Matt. 26:39). There was a part of Him that did not want to go to the cross, but this unwillingness was not going to stop Him from doing what the Father asked and trusting Him for the promise set before Him.

In scripture, we find a loving Father that desires us to not be like an unwilling stubborn animal, but rather He desires that we draw near to Him!

I will instruct you and teach you in the way in which you should go; I will counsel you with My eye upon you. Do not be as the horse or as the mule which have no understanding, whose trappings include bit and bridle to hold them in check, otherwise they will not come near to you.

Psalm 32:8–9

Hardness of Heart

Perhaps the biggest hindrance to moving forward is a hard heart. This can be likened to stubbornness. But I think it goes deeper than that into the very part of our souls that doubts and questions in an untrusting manner.

The Bible uses this phrase to describe people like the Pharisees, who in Jesus' time did not trust Jesus. They questioned the good things He did, like telling a man to pick up his pallet and walk, forgiveness of sins, healing the blind, the man with the shriveled hand, and feeding the thousands.

A hard heart is not impressionable or willing to change, adapt, or receive. Similar to hardened clay, a hard heart cannot be molded. The prophet Jeremiah was led to a Potter's house to watch him and the

LORD spoke these words, "*'Can I not, O house of Israel, deal with you as this potter does?' declares the* LORD" (*Jeremiah* 18:6).

A precious scripture in Proverbs states, *"Give me your heart, my son; And let your eyes delight in my ways"* (23:26). God desires to have our heart and care for it Himself.

Defensiveness

In moving forward, I also noticed a defensiveness towards the idea of having children. When someone would ask, "Do you have children? Why not?" The answer springs back in a sharp defensive remark, "It's up to God."

There is a defensive part of our heart that thinks, *I really can't move forward, not unless God is surely going to make this little one live.*

I almost felt defensive towards my own thinking about children. I would shun the thoughts away and try to focus on something else. As with bitterness and hardness of heart, God is looking in our souls and desiring there to be an openness, a willingness, despite the walls we may put up.

Dear Lord, in moving forward I face my own hard heart, my unwillingness to be vulnerable and open. Help me where I am defensive, keep my heart moldable and lead me on to Your best.

Timing

When is it the right time to have a baby? We say this in today's society like it is all up to us; to some extent it is, and to another it is not. In some cases, like artificial insemination, this may be so. It's funny that when you have a miscarriage or problems conceiving, one must ask, "How much control do I really have over this?"

In the Bible, timing is very important to God. This is not the kind of time that is twenty-four hours in a day, rather the kind of time that unravels the mysteries of God in a divine setting. This is God's time (kairos in the Greek). Sarah, Abraham's wife, was to have a child in God's timing. To her, His timing must have seemed ridiculous. She was ninety years old. Certainly that was not the "right" timing. Or so she thought. She laughed at the promise. "And the LORD said to Abraham, 'Why did Sarah laugh, saying, "Shall I indeed bear a child, when I am so old?" Is anything to difficult for the LORD? At the *appointed time* I will return to you, at this time next year, and Sarah will have a son'" (Gen. 18:13–14). "At the appointed time," He said. God did it. "So Sarah conceived and bore a son to Abraham in his old age, *at the appointed time* of which God had spoken to him" (Gen. 21:2). He brought laughter out of the whole thing. When I ponder this story, I am struck with awe. His ways really are higher than our ways (Isa. 55:8–9). It is miraculous. They have a testimony that has lived on for years.

Did you ever stop to think about the conditions of the time that you were born in? Did you ever think, *Maybe I was born in the wrong generation?* Or do you think about what your parents were going through? It is amazing to think that if you were conceived on a different day, you would be a totally different person. If one sperm in a million had been different, you would have been a different person. You are who you are because of God's timing and miraculous design.

We operate on time (chronos). We have alarm clocks and schedules that depict our every hour. We set our time to wake up and our time to sleep. We try to keep to these numbers and sometimes cut people off driving for this time. There are certain things in life that do not seem to operate on this time: plants, buses, and some animals. If someone interrupts "our" time, we call it "bad timing." Was it good timing for them?

There are things that seem urgent, but what makes them so urgent? Is it time? Man's time is not God's time. He will sometimes nudge us to talk to someone in need, even though we have a schedule to keep! He isn't watching us and expecting us to come spend time with Him at exactly 6:30 PM. He does have set times. But He isn't controlled by it. God knows our "bio-logical" clocks are ticking, but He is not stressed. He can take a beaten down old, barren "clock" like Sarah's and wind it back up, and place it on a shelf for all to see. Sometimes I think He likes to do that. <u>He takes things that are broken and weak and makes them beautiful masterpieces.</u> Do you ever wonder why He bothers with us? He is producing in us an eternal glory that outweighs the physical.

The psalmist David wrote, "*My times are in Your hand*" (*Ps.* 31:15). He may have written this in a cave waiting for the promise to be fulfilled that he would be king. He trusted that in God's time he would be. In the same way, we can trust our times are in His hand.

"*Trying Again*"

After wrestling with the issues that trying again brings up, then comes the plunge! Note that I wrote "trying" again in quotations. Because after experiencing loss in this area, it is evident that God has to be involved in the process. You and your spouse need to walk through this step with prayer and sense of peace with God about whatever the outcome may be.

It is also important not to let lovemaking become a ritual act of reproduction. This can put a lot of stress on both parties to try to make it happen! You and your spouse may need to communicate and take extra time to romance one another.

A child is the outcome of your love. When you do conceive, it will then be out of a loving and memorable time that you shared.

In this process, it is important to be sensitive to your emotions and for your spouse to be aware of that you are choosing to make yourself vulnerable and open.

Waiting for the Outcome

Then comes the waiting! Sometimes a month can go by so slowly! As you wait, bring Him your thoughts and worries. Reading scripture helps to take your mind off wondering if you are or are not pregnant. I found it helpful to try to live life as normal. I had been so cautious and fearful thinking *But what if I am pregnant?* It was helpful for me to disregard those thoughts and replace them with thoughts of trust. *God will sustain it if I am.*

It was freeing to realize I would have to trust Him either way! Trust Him to keep the life of the baby or to go through the steps again.

For some women, it may take awhile to conceive again. It can be a long agonizing waiting period, or it can be a chance to draw close to God and learn to run to Him as you wait on Him and trust Him. He is using this time to test our hearts and to bring us closer to Him.

Other women may conceive right away, but the thoughts and agony of whether or not this life will make it can be just as unbearable as waiting.

Keep Hope Alive

It is very helpful in the waiting season to keep hope alive. God's promise to us as we wait is, "*Those who wait (hope in) for the Lord will gain new strength; they will mount up with wings like eagles, they will run and not get tired, they will walk and not become weary*" (*Isaiah* 40:31).

Waiting and hoping are active ways to trust God and draw strength from Him to keep going. Hope is an expectation that God "is." That He is real and does know the circumstances that surround us. Hope that we will see Him in heaven and see Him work in this current age.

The Psalms are filled with encouraging words that help to keep hope alive.

"And now, LORD, for what do I wait? My hope is in You." Psalm 38:7

"For I hope in You, O LORD; You will answer, O LORD my God." Psalm 39:15

"For You are my hope; O LORD God, You are
my confidence from my youth."

Psalm 71:5

Hope is a mystery similar to love. It is delicate
and precious. God is referred to as a God of Hope,
"Now may the God of hope fill you with all joy and
peace in believing, so that you will abound in hope by
the power of the Holy Spirit" Romans 15:13

Through Jesus, we are all given a living hope,
a hope that carries us to eternal life.
Blessed be the God and Father of our LORD
Jesus Christ, who according to His great
mercy has caused us to be a born again to a
living hope through the resurrection of Jesus
Christ from the dead, to obtain an inheritance
which is imperishable and undefiled and will
not fade away, reserved in heaven for you.

1 Peter 1:3–4

He has given us hope beyond this life, and it is
not a hope that is dead now but rather a living hope.
It is vital, as with most living things, to sustain and
nurture your hope in God and keep it alive.

It is easy to give way to the enemy and fall into a
state of hopelessness. Perhaps the best way to guard
against hopelessness is to "sanctify [set apart] Christ

as LORD in your hearts" (1 Peter 3:15). This means to let Him be the one who keeps your heart. As Master of your heart, He will help you stand up against the enemy and defend the hope that is in you. If you are in a hopeless state of being, still give Him your heart. He is able to plant hope again in your heart.

In order to guard against a false sense of hope, it helps to put your hope solely in God and not in the outcome of circumstances. Here is a simple prayer for and of hope:

Dear Father, thank You for being a God of hope. Thank You that You are able to give me hope again. Hope that You are real and that You will be with me no matter the circumstance. Lord, I place my hope in You and not in circumstances. Forgive me for the times I lose heart and live in hopelessness instead of having living hope. I thank You, Jesus, most of all for the hope of eternal life for that is the greatest gift!

Trusting in God Is a Lifestyle

Once you are able to wait on the LORD and have a sense of hope, it is important to learn that <u>trusting God is a lifestyle</u>. It is not a one-time deal; this is perhaps one of the hardest lessons to learn.

Trust does not come easily to us as people because we have been hurt throughout our lives. We learn not to trust people or anything, simply from people, society, and circumstances. When these fail us, we blame God as though He is the untrustworthy one.

But now more than ever, as you move forward and take steps of vulnerability, it is vital to trust God.

No Other Option But to Trust

I quickly realized during my third pregnancy that there simply was no other option but to trust Him for the outcome. Either way, I'd have trust. I had to trust that He would carry this pregnancy through to completion. It was a day-by-day trust of relying completely on His mercy. I knew with each day that passed I would also have to trust Him, if perhaps I would lose this one too. I would have to trust that He would carry me through as He had done the other times.

I took comfort in the fact that either way His promise to me was to carry me.

> You have been borne by Me from birth and have been carried from the womb, even to your old age I will be the same, and even to your graying years I will bear you! I have done it, and I will carry you; I will bear you and I will deliver you.
>
> Is. 46:3–4

God promised Israel to carry them, and I believe He extends this promise for us today.

Trusting Despite Circumstances

"But even if He does not..."
Daniel 3:18

Shadrach, Meshach, and Abednego replied to the king, "O Nebuchadnezzar, we do not need to give you an answer concerning this matter. If it be so, our God whom we serve is able to deliver us from the furnace of blazing fire; and He will deliver us out of your hand, O King. But even if He does not, let it be known to you, O king, that we are not going to serve your gods or worship the golden image that you have set up." (Daniel 3:16–18).

Though the fig tree should not blossom and there be no fruit on the vines, though the yield of the olive should fail and the fields produce no food. Though the flock should be cut off from the fold and there be no cattle in the stalls, Yet I will exult in the LORD, I will rejoice in the God of my salvation.

Habakkuk 3:17–18

Sometimes it's hard to trust God because He often allows us to go through some pretty crazy things. He let the disciples strain at the oars before coming to them on the water. He let Shadrach, Meshach, and Abednego be thrown into flames. Daniel was left for dead in a lion's den. Trusting God does not mean the absence of pain or chaos.

Really it makes no sense to logically trust in these circumstances. It's easy to trust God when life is going well and all our prayers are being answered. But what about when there is no fruit on the vine, "no cattle in the stalls," if something should fail? I don't know about you, but if someone were going to throw me in a burning furnace, I don't know if I'd have the guts that those three had. They were devoted to God despite everything. And they trusted that even if God let them be thrown in the fire, they could still follow. I don't know what scares me more, the burning furnace or following God who let them be thrown in!

In God's defense however, He did meet them in the midst of the fire and deliver them with out any harm being done to their bodies,

> Then Shadrach, Meshach, and Abednego came out of the midst of the fire. The satraps, prefects, the governors, and the king's high officials gathered around and saw in regard to these men that the fire had no effect on the bodies of these men nor was the hair of their head singed, nor were

their trousers damaged, nor had the smell of
fire even come upon them.

Daniel 3:26–27

Not even a hair burned. Amazing. I can't even
blow dry my hair without getting a hair burnt here
and there. God did intervene. But it was not as simple as "not going through the fire." Yes, He did allow
them to get thrown into a burning furnace, but He
chose to be there with them (vs. 25) and in the end
bring them up without harm.

It's hard for me to trust despite the circumstances.
I am affected by my surroundings, what I see, what I
hear, what's going on. I can't escape it. I have to make
a conscious choice to trust Him even though what I
may be seeing is really discouraging.

Moving forward and trusting God takes that kind
of faith. Faith that walks not by sight, but by believing *He is.* He is God even if the circumstances don't
change. Even if I'm thrown in the fire or the stalls
are empty.

God may lead us to continue to *act* in trust, even
if there is nothing that *confirms* or seems to affirm
this is the right direction. Keep building that boat,
Noah; it might rain some day. Take another spin
around Jericho; the walls just might fall down. Keep
trying; you may be expecting an Isaac some day. Trust
despite the circumstances.

Dear Lord, I place my trust in You and Your promise to carry me. I choose today to trust You despite my circumstances. I choose to act on my trust and follow even if You don't answer.

Peace and Eternity

Great Day in Heaven
By: Koa Siu

I have never seen you, but I know your name
The joy and expectancy of waiting for your time
made my heart overflow
For you I cried, and happiness filled my eyes
when I heard that you were coming
For you my heart died,
or came about as close as I could get
knowing you were gone

And I don't think I will ever understand
why you were taken away so soon
But I'll find my peace in the hope of the day
When I hear my name behind me, turn around to see
And not too far away a man is walking up to me

Though I've never seen his face,
I have loved him all his life
It'll be a great day in heaven,
when I see my son for the first time

I wonder what you'll tell me,
I wonder what I'll say, standing face to face
I'll be new to heaven so I guess you'll
show me the way
around where you've been living always

Maybe then I will start to understand
why you were taken away so soon
And I'll find my peace in the hope of the day

When I'll hear my name behind me,
turn around to see
And not too far away you're there walking up to me
Though I've never seen your face,
I have loved you all your life
It'll be a great day in heaven,
when I see you son for the first time

And everything will be brand new,
and I will look back with satisfaction
At all the things He's brought me through
And there will be peace, and there will be love,

and there will be
freedom and hope and joy
and there will be you! Oh you...

And we'll hear my name behind me,
we'll turn around to see
And you will introduce me
to the man who's walking up to me
Though I've never seen His face,
He has loved me all my life
It'll be a great day in heaven,
when I see my Savior,
And I meet my son for the first time

Download this song for free at
www.runtoyou.org

"...for the kingdom of heaven belongs to such as these."
Matthew 19:14

My husband wrote a beautiful song after our first
miscarriage that spoke of seeing our son in heaven
when he gets there. At first, I thought it sounded
lovely, but instead of wrapping my arms around him
and letting it touch my heart, I questioned him about
its theology! I didn't like the song because I just
didn't know if it was true. Was this little lost one with

Jesus in eternity? Would he really be someone when I got to heaven? Some time has passed since he wrote that song, and now I find it does touch me because of the peace I've found that this precious life is in His hands and He doesn't turn away children. Jesus made a point to embrace children and teach others to be more childlike. He took them in His arms and blessed them (Mark 9:16). Scripture says, "*The kingdom of heaven belongs to such as these.*"

Beth Moore writes about these verses,

> As I see the tenderness Christ held in His heart for children, I wonder sometimes if He did not consider time spent with children as the closest thing to heaven on earth!...I also believe this verse substantiates what most of us have believed by faith; children who die go to heaven. If He received them so readily while on this earth because of the tenderness of His heart, how could He possibly bar their entrance to the very kingdom He described them as representing? To do so would be completely contrary to His character.
>
> Living Beyond Yourself, 144

Heaven belongs to children. It's where they reside and where we are called to have the same heart in order to enter as well.

Truly I say to you, unless you are converted
and become like children, you will not enter
the kingdom of heaven. Whoever then hum-
bles himself as this child, he is the greatest in
the kingdom of heaven. And whoever receives
one such child in My name receives Me.

Matthew 18:3–5

He Knows Them

You may have heard an older song, *"He knows my
name, before even time began, my life was in His hands."*
Scripture gives us examples of God's foreknowledge
for the unborn.

"Listen to Me, O islands, and pay attention
you peoples from afar. The LORD called Me
from the womb; from the body of My mother
He named Me." Isaiah 49:1

"Before I formed you in the womb I knew
you, And before you were born I consecrated
you; I have appointed you a prophet to the
nations."

Jeremiah 1:5

"For you formed my inward parts; You wove me in my mother's womb. I will give thanks to You, for I am fearfully and wonderfully made; wonderful are Your works, and my soul knows it very well. My frame was not hidden from You, When I was made in secret and skillfully wrought in the depths of the earth; Your eyes have seen my unformed substance; and in Your book were all written the days that were ordained for me when as yet there was not one of them."

Psalm 139:13–16

God has a plan and knows them by name. This can be so reassuring when suffering from the loss of miscarriage. We may not know them. We may not even get to see them. But we can rest assured that someone does. He knows every hair on our head. He knows what we are thinking before a word is formed. And He knows who we are before we are even knit together.

David can't fathom it, "Such knowledge is too wonderful for me" (Psalm 139:6). God knew David before he was born. Jeremiah was appointed from the womb. John the Baptist responded to the Spirit at the presence of Jesus in the womb.

My little ones may not have been great biblical

characters or raised their hands in the pews or said the sinner's prayer, but I can trust that God knew him and her while still in the womb. He is the one to determine where they will be in eternity. Like Enoch, God may have simply taken them.

Somehow these little ones have a direct link to the Father. Jesus describes it this way, "*See that you do not despise one of these little ones, for I say to you that their angels in heaven continually see the face of My Father who is in heaven. For the Son of Man has come to save that which is lost*" (Matthew 18:10–11). It's as though there is something so special to God about children that He is constantly checking in on them.

These little ones are truly a treasure and their passing matters to Him. "*Precious in the sight of the Lord is the death of His godly ones*" (Psalm 116:15). The New Living Translation reads, "*The Lord cares deeply when His loved ones die.*"

In closing, I want to encourage you that He is a refuge for them. "*The eternal God is a dwelling place, and underneath are the everlasting arms*" (Deuteronomy 33:27). In His arms, there *is* peace and eternity.

Dear Father, thank You for keeping and caring about these little ones. I thank You for Your peace that surpasses understanding. Thank You for Your everlasting arms that hold them. You remain the eternal God who is a dwelling place for those we've lost.

Bibliography

The Holy Bible. *Updated New American Standard Bible. Grand Rapids, Michigan: Zondervan Publishing,* 1999.

Eareckson Tada, Joni. *When God Weeps, Why Our Sufferings Matter to the Almighty.*
Grand Rapids, Michigan: Zondervan Publishing, 1997.

Moore, Beth. *Living Beyond Yourself, Exploring the Fruit of the Spirit.* Nashville, Tennessee: LifeWay Press, 1998.

Sittser, Jerry. *A Grace Disguised: How the Soul Grows through Loss.* Grand Rapids, Michigan: Zondervan Publishing, 1995.

Made in the USA
Lexington, KY
30 May 2016